I0414918

This Journal Belongs To

____

www.ingramcontent.com/pod-product-compliance
Lightning Source LLC
Chambersburg PA
CBHW072057280526
45788CB00006B/2317
9781093403275